Speaking Skin

Howard Coleman Jr

Acknowledgements

First and foremost, I would like thank God for restoring my peace of mind and healing my broken heart. Thank you Lord for rescuing me from drowning in a sea of depression and self-hate.

I would like to thank you mother, Barbara, for always listening to me. No matter how frustrated I became, you were always willing to offer me words of encouragement. You showed me the love that sometimes I was unwilling to give to myself.

I would like to thank you dad, Howard Sr., for always inspiring me to achieve my goals in life and being available whenever I needed you. You were always present for every event that mattered in my life.

I would like to thank you sister, Katarsha, for helping me to develop a more positive image of myself. You were my only friend during my early childhood years when no one else volunteered to be.

I'm so grateful to my cousin Wenona for being so understanding every time I called during my many nights of tears and sorrow. My grandma Lottie for speaking her mind, always putting a smile on my face and keeping me company on the porch.

I'm thankful for having my friend Jacinta

in my life during my high school days. Jacinta you stood up for me when others criticized me, and I truly appreciate you.

Thank you Oprah Winfrey for being an inspiration and empowering me to make necessary changes in my life.

Speaking Skin

Copyright © 2010 by Howard Coleman Jr

Introduction

If your skin could speak, what would it
say? Or maybe your skin is silent and
doesn't need to speak at all. But if your
skin is anything like mine, it isn't happy;
my skin reminds me daily of how unsatisfied
it is. As a matter of fact, it won't keep
quiet and creates enough noise that others
tell me to do something about it. But what
do you do when you're making the best
choices with what you know and your best
just isn't producing results well enough
for yourself or anyone else?

People may say "celebrate your uniqueness
or differences". But honestly, there are
times when you just want to blend in and
not stand out. If you are receiving
compliments or praise for your differences,
that's one thing. But if you are being

ridiculed or put down because of those differences, that doesn't call for a celebration. That's not a good feeling.

People may trivialize it and say "your skin isn't that bad; you're making a big deal out of nothing." However, on us, acne, freckles, wrinkles, moles, or scars may not seem that bad, but if it were to show up on their face, trust me they'll have a change of heart.

Sometimes, people may even say it's all in our head. However, if you spend minutes to hours trying to correct or cover up problem areas with your face, the problem is no longer imagined but real. When people frown or squint their eyes as they stare at you, you soon realize that others see your skin as a problem as well. When you've been hearing all your life from people, magazines, books, and television that smooth and flawless is what makes someone beautiful and you don't fit that description, you feel unattractive. However, sometimes you just have to learn how to reject certain information, especially if hearing it makes you feel worse about yourself.

People say "what doesn't kill you will make you stronger". However, that's not always the case. Some experiences can weaken your spirit and force you to question your own existence. I spent years trying to figure out where I belonged. Being teased continuously, I felt like I had been kicked out of humanity. I took on their cruel comments as proof that something was really wrong with me.

When you encounter unwanted changes to

your skin whether it be wrinkles, moles, acne, you may ask "wait a minute, where did this come from, why is it here, and when will it go away? It's a mystery to you, but it's a mystery you are determined to uncover. The impact on your self-esteem depends on at what point in your life it happens, the intensity of it, and how long those pimples last? Acne breakouts can be highly unpredictable and hard to master. Some skin care products can help but at times your skin can throw a curveball and will break out underneath those skin care ointments and creams. Sometimes your skin problems seem to frustrate the most experienced doctors. They don't know what to do and get irritated because the creams or pills they're prescribing aren't producing desired results.

I often asked myself "what did I do so horrific in my early childhood to deserve this?" Sometimes I feel like I am on an emotional see-saw where my confidence goes up and down depending on the condition of my skin. I asked myself "how did I get this but most importantly, how can I make it disappear? " You may consider skin break outs as a phase in life you don't want to talk about but still hoping to move through it as quickly as possible.

The question now becomes "what are we able to do about it?" Are we going to take in the criticism and allow it to strip us of our self-esteem? Or are we going use these adverse situations to empower ourselves? Skin problems shows up in every race, gender, and various age groups. Trust me, you're not alone. My wish is that my painful past/present experiences

can comfort you in the present and offer

renewed hope for your future.

Poetry

<u>Poem 1</u>

Life can seem so unfair

About my troubles, no one seems to care

The ridicule I receive from others never

ceases

To break my self-esteem into bits and

pieces

Some relatives and friends joke about my

sadness

Telling me to get over this madness

Around others, happiness can no longer be

faked

My birth has got to be a mistake

I'm trying my best

But society's insults can my stomach no

longer digest

I must conclude

That all I have to look forward to is a

life of solitude

<u>Poem 2</u>

I arrive at the airport with confidence

Hoping others wouldn't notice that my bumps

were so immense

But as soon as I board the plane

All those stares are about to drive me

insane

I am trying to find someone else with bad

skin

So this awful feeling of loneliness

wouldn't come back again

I hear giggles as I pass through the aisles

I feel dizzy as though I've been walking

for miles

Everyone keeps glancing with disapproval at

my bumps

I feel like unwanted trash that belongs in

a dump

Poem 3

I decided to go to a teen party tonight

I hope the DJ doesn't turn on the lights

Because I don't want others to see my

hideous skin

But to my surprise even with the lights

off, I was picked on once again

They laugh at me because I am so thin

Feeling embarrassed, I lower my chin

Feeling like an outcast, I leave the dance

floor

I don't feel like being an annoyance to

others anymore

But as I sit, I look to my right appalled

at first sight

At my own reflection in the mirror, I was

filled with fright

<u>Poem 4</u>

People can be so cruel and mean

Ridiculing my face and lowering my self

esteem

Around the house I continue to mope

Giving up all hope

That my skin will become clear

My faith disappears each time I look into

the mirror

In addition to acne, I have moles

HELP!! I'm turning into a troll

<u>Poem 5</u>

I try my hardest to be a man

To bottle my feelings once more can my

heart no longer withstand?

How can this be?

Everyone else appears to be good looking

but me

The rest of the world dislikes me because

of my ugly appearance

I'm sure my school wouldn't be saddened if

I pulled a sudden disappearance

Right about now, I need a friend

Someone to be there with me through the

thick and thin

Picking me up when these skin problems wear

me down

However, as I look around

I realize there is no such friend to be

found

<u>Poem 6</u>

During the last days of class, I am hoping

someone wants to take my picture

But of course, no one wants a photo of an

ugly creature

I walk around hoping to be included

But the classmates form small circles, all

of which I am excluded

I feel like an outcast once again

Believing their response is because of the

eruption of bumps on my skin

Tears are about to fall from my weary eyes

I want to tell them all good-bye

I wait for about 15 minutes after class

However they just continued to walk pass

I try to keep my cool

But I feel like such a fool

<u>Poem 7</u>

None of these acne medications work

For the cure of acne my mind continues to

search

But every time I turn around, excess oil

lurks underneath my skin

Causing acne breakouts once again

The dermatologist put me on a pill

I believe my skin will finally heal

I take the pills each night

However my face continues to be a gruesome

sight

I dislike myself now more than ever

I'm destined to live life as an ugly

monster forever

I become desperate and lose hope

I burst the bumps and dry them with harsh

ivory soap

While rinsing, the water feels like acid

giving me a burning sensation

I scream out in complete frustration

Afterwards, I then look into the mirror

Hoping my skin will be a tad bit clearer

Dang, nothing has changed

My bumps still remain

<u>Poem 8</u>

I go to the barbershop

Even here, my self-esteem drops

My barber keeps asking me why I don't

control my acne

I then realize my acne doesn't just affect

me

It irritates everybody else around me

He can't even cut my hair because my skin

distracts him

The chances of my skin ever going unnoticed

becomes more slim

Frustrated, he rubs on my skin a handful of

alcohol

Seeing the results, he isn't satisfied at

all

He then takes matters in his own hands

The sight of my persistent acne could he no

longer withstand

He squeezes my bumps with his hands that

are covered with grease

I sit in silence hoping this physical

torment would cease

He now makes bursting my bumps his biweekly

routine

Which makes it more unlikely for my self-

worth to ever be redeemed.

<u>Poem 9</u>

I woke up this morning filled with good

cheer

Until I look in the mirror and resembled

Rudolf the red nose reindeer

In class students continue to glance over

at me

It's obvious they can't control their

curiosity

They stare at me like I've committed an

unforgivable sin

Showing my face in public again!

Poem 10

My sullen spirit is longing for a

resurrection

When will my life take a turn in a positive

direction?

When will it be my time to shine?

Instead of always experiencing dramatic

self-esteem declines

Poem 11

This year things have changed

I no longer looked the same

Clearer skin has given me a feeling of

pride

In public, my face is no longer what I have

to hide

They aren't so quick to talk about me

Which fills my heart with glee

I no longer think of my skin as a disgrace

22

Self-hatred is slowly being erased.

Thoughts and Experiences

I would prefer to walk along the walls in the hallway instead of walking in the middle in high school. Oftentimes, I would be forced to walk in the middle. It was torturous to have students look at the left and right sides of my face.

One of my classmates in my history class had a pimple form on his nose. It lasted for about two weeks. I couldn't help but glance at his pimple every now and then. I would check out my nose out in the mirror often. Then as his pimple was fading into nonexistence, a pimple on my nose was forming. It was gigantic and persisted for about 2 months. How is this possible? Is acne airborne now? Good grief!

When playing sports, I got hit with the

ball by accident. I was a nervous wreck.
Do you know how dirty that sports equipment
is? As soon as the game ended, I rushed to
the restroom to rinse my face off.

Also, someone suggested I get a tattoo.
I replied, thanks but no thanks. I already
have plenty of shapes, sizes, colors and
designs on my face; it's called having
combination skin. I don't need additional
marks.

I heard often growing up that all teens
get acne. I disagree; I have been in
plenty of classrooms as a high school
student and was the only one with bumps on
my face. That myth can set kids up to feel
even worse about themselves.

Having one or two real friends helped
having skin problems much more pleasant
because they listened & cared. I could talk

about how I felt about my skin, and my feelings of sadness when my face would break out. I discussed the products I was using, and how they helped or worsened my skin. We would offer compliments to each other about our physical appearances. We never put each other down. It was okay to feel insecure amongst each other.

While volunteering as a tutor, one child said "why is your face so oily". Kids can say some of the rudest comments at times. It's not easy trying not to take what they say personal. Most of those kids lack insight and don't realize how what they're saying is making you feel. I just politely got up, wiped my face with a damp paper towel and continued to help them with their work.

There was a commercial that marketed a

machine that would fix skins problems. It
would use a needle that would pick your
skin and extract the pimple. I was so
excited about that product because of the
way it was promoted. I was desperate and
was willing to try anything to improve my
skin. I didn't have any money so I had to
depend on my parents to purchase it for me.
My mom said "no" once she found out the
product was a machine using a needle. I
was furious and said "you must want me to
be ugly. If you love me, you would want me
to be happy". As teens, we may try to
manipulate our parents to get what we want.
I had put a lot of hope into that product
and disappointments are very painful. She
could have just ordered it to shut me up.
However, she didn't waver in her decision,
and I'm glad she didn't. She did what was

best for me, not what was easiest for her.
I would have scarred and scratched my face
up with that needle. I haven't seen that
product in years; it was taken off the
market just as quickly as it was put on it.

I would attend community events that
were video recorded. I would try my best to
look away from the camera, or put a hand
over my face or head. If I saw a
photographer, I would say to myself "that
person better not be taking my picture".
Plus, bright lights are not my friend. I
preferred dimmed lighting in that
auditorium. I had a question for the
speaker but I was surely not about to shift
unwanted gazes towards me.

During class, my teacher decided to talk
about steroids and how they can
consequently result in individuals

developing acne. I felt so embarrassed. I
wasn't using them but definitely appeared
to be experiencing the side effects.

At work, my supervisor called me into
his office and asked "what do you think
causes your acne?" I suspected I had the
most severe acne amongst all the employees
but now it's being confirmed. So not only
am I being evaluated on my performance and
productivity, but now I'm being judged on
my physical appearance. He continued to
discuss solutions for my skin problem even
when another co-worker walked in. How
embarrassing! At this point, I'm feeling
overwhelmed. Every time I report to work,
I'm wondering if the condition of my skin
meets his approval.

I disliked standing up on a crowded bus
shuttle, especially while all eyes seemed

to be focused on me. It was awful when passengers had nothing better to do than stare at my face. They weren't talking on the phone, talking to each other, or reading. Those were nerve wrecking experiences, and I felt I was going to pass out at times.

My skin's condition would be reflected in my attire at work. Clear days, I felt confident and would wear dress shirt, dress pants and ties. On bad days, I felt drained and didn't want to stand out. I would wear a collared shirt and khakis.

I'm dreading my approaching birthday because I know my co-workers are going to give me a cake. That's the last thing I need. I hope they don't expect me to eat it!

One co-worker offered me a chocolate

candy bar. My thoughts were "Hello, do you not see my skin? You must really dislike me."

New pimples, can I please get rid of the old ones first!

Some days I felt mighty low, but I promised   myself I would keep my head up.

In high school, prom was approaching. My skin looked awful. I was using prescription medication, and it still looked terrible. I had so many scars and acne. The disapproving facial expression on my date and her father's face when I arrived was disheartening. We decided to go with two other classmates and their dates. At the dinner table, everyone else had flawless skin. Initially, I felt awkward and out of place. However, my sense of

humor made me feel more at ease. This is
my night; there is no need for me to feel
down and out about something I can't change
at the moment. I'll make the best of this
worst case scenario. I had a wonderful
time. No one brought the skin problem to
my attention so I'm definitely not going to
bring it to their attention. I'm not a
fool. As we entered into the prom, it was
very dim. I felt confident. Most
importantly, the pictures turned out great.
The pictures made me look fantastic. A
tragic beginning turned into a happy
ending.

A teacher remarked how men/women
breakout in the face with one or two
pimples when they're getting married. Well
what's your explanation for me having 5-10
pimples and no wedding?

At times, I found myself jumping in a pool, submerging my face underwater hoping to come up with flawless skin. Oftentimes, I drifted into a trance, but the shortness of breath forced me to break out of it. The chlorinated water did not help but dried my face out. My skin produced even more oil to hydrate my skin and then it later broke out even more.

There have been days when my face had bumps resembling volcanoes and hills. The hills were the worst ones, and toughest to pop. Pimples in sensitive areas on your face such as your ears, lips, eyebrows hurt worse when popped.

I was playing sports, and I remember one guy calling a girl crater face. I wonder what he's calling me after I walk off the court.

I had to take a blood thinning medication for deep vein thrombosis which caused a blood clot in my leg. While on the blood thinning medication, my face didn't heal as fast after I popped a pimple. As a result, scabs would just sit there. Sometimes I would smile and oil would come out. I had to get off that medication as soon as possible because I could not concentrate at work while my face was bleeding and oozing out oil.

When I was 14yrs old, I dreamed I would grow out of my acne once I turned 20yrs old because of what I was told; it was just a phase teens go thru. However, my 20s rolled around and I still have it. I cried and experienced intense grief for being forced to let go of a dream that didn't come true, well not for me. Having your dreams shattered to pieces can be very painful.

In high school, I was late for class at least 40 days during the school year. My mom or dad always sent a note stating "I was late because I was sick" so I could be excused. However, the truth was I was indeed sick, not in my body, but in my mind. I was depressed and stressed trying to correct my skin so I could at least look decent.

I truly prefer driving in a car with a tint. There was a sense of security gained from having a tint over my windows because I knew people couldn't see me clearly. However, when I would drive a rental car with no tint, I felt so exposed. I would sometimes see the damaged skin of other drivers with no car tint so I'm sure others could see mine.

There were times I disliked walking through the parking lot. They were too many cars with so many windows that displayed my reflection. Some cars made me look stunning and attractive while a few portrayed me as looking unattractive.

Sometimes people with problematic skin can be very insensitive. An advisor at my college told me after reading one of my poems, "it's just acne, no big deal". His skin wasn't clear at all, and I was shocked that he was so insensitive. That just reminded me that people can share common problems, but their experiences can vary greatly. Very few people understood the depths of my pain, humiliation, or despair.

I used to wear colored contacts to divert the attention off my skin to my eyes. People were too busy trying to figure out if that was my real eye color or not instead of focusing on the spots on my skin. I realized I couldn't wear them forever, even if they are extended wear. It got to the point that I didn't think I looked good without them. I'm sure those that wear makeup can identify with how I felt. Those contacts have to come out eventually just like the makeup has to be washed off. I have to love myself as I am with all of my glories and faults; however, it hasn't always been easy.

There was a point in my life when I just didn't have the money to pay for those over the counter or prescription skin care products. I also didn't have the health insurance to see a dermatologist. At that point, I became afraid and thought I couldn't make it without them. I had to go for about 5 months without products. Unexpectedly, my skin looked great and felt healthier. That happened to be one of the best decisions in my life. That's when I realized, I didn't need to rely on them as much. I do not wish to be dependent on taking acne treatments every day for the rest of my life. I had to find a natural cure that works for me. I just try to avoid eating too many sweets, dairy products, or greasy food. I drink plenty of water, get plenty of rest, exercise, and avoid becoming too stressed out. However, I do prefer to have acne medications just on standby in case of emergencies. If you are experiencing a great amount of stress, then you just might need the additional help that those products can offer you temporarily.

Sometimes my skin itched really badly, like mosquito bites all on my face. That typically happened when new pimples were just forming, and I was dreading their arrival.

Taking a shower was not always a soothing or relaxing experience. That water felt like a knife ripping my skin apart, especially after I just popped a pimple.

Sometimes I pretended to be on the phone if I was walking through a crowd of people. I needed to shield the left and right sides of my face from public scrutiny and unwanted stares.

When it gets really hot and you're riding in the car with a group of others and the windows are down, your face may become so oily and itchy. I had to continuously wipe my face on my shirt during those road trips. It's okay to politely ask them to turn on the air conditioning in the car because the heat from outdoors is making you feel uncomfortable.

Sometimes medications would dry my face out, and I'd have to scrape off the dead skin. Those dry patches would take days to go away on their own. I felt better without having dry patches on my face.

My parents told me they both had acne growing up. At first, I felt as though I was doomed after hearing that news. However, knowing this allowed me to understand why I was suffering with it so I felt I had some type of closure. However, genetics isn't going stop me from finding a solution for it. I refuse to get into that mindset of feeling destined to suffer with acne for the rest of my life and that I have no control over my fate. I have the power shape my present and future and so do you.

Sometimes, I thought I got out all of the oil after a few pinches and be able to walk out in public. However, I soon realized some bumps were still oozing oil out on my face and sometimes dried up without me noticing. So make sure you glance in the mirror several minutes after you have recently adjusted your skin.

Have you ever popped a pimple and it decreased in size only temporarily? However, a day or two later, that same pimple grows back with a vengeance. It seemed like an endless cycle and can be so frustrating.

I've tried microdermabrasion, and
that procedure was physically painful.
That machine stayed glued on my nose trying
to suck out the oil. The following day
scabs formed, and scars were all over my
face. My face looked awful. To make
matters worse, I went to a restaurant two
days later. As I was walking in, I crossed
paths with someone that teased me
relentlessly growing up. When you see an
arch enemy from childhood, you want to look
your best. However, that wasn't the case
with me. We greeted each other but I
intentionally kept that conversation short.
I was not about to give that individual the
time to tear my self-esteem apart.

The lighting in the gym depended on
the time of day. I preferred to go the
evening. I'm able to focus on my workout

than being preoccupied with my face. I
can't concentrate on my workout in the
morning and afternoon because it's so
bright in there, and my skin's defects look
amplified in all those mirrors.

Before a performance with my dance
group in college, my group members wanted
me to put on make-up. I respectfully
declined. They thought I was being
difficult, but I knew my skin wouldn't be
pleased with that decision. Twenty minutes
in the spotlight on stage was not worth 2
weeks or more of a hideous disfigurement on
my face.

During my senior year, someone said I
had the bone structure to be a model. I
said to myself, "yeah right, do you not see
my broken skin that would disqualify me?"

When friends use your restroom, they

oftentimes try to use your skin care products leisurely for one pimple while you may have a face full. They may use it as a luxury item while we need it for social survival.

I got so upset when I was reading the newspaper as Valentine's Day was approaching. The article stated how chocolate can improve your skin because of certain ingredients. Companies will publish anything claiming it's medically proven to sell a product. Don't be fooled, reflect on your experiences. Every time I ate chocolate, my face broke out. They claim chocolate doesn't break individuals out. Yeah, if they have clear skin chances of their face ever breaking out is pretty slim. But if you have skin like mine, I would advise you to leave it alone.

Growing up reading fairytales and novels, the villain was normally characterized as having bumpy or blemished skin. Even in cartoons, the witch had moles or lumps on her face and described as ugly. The hero was described as attractive with smooth skin. Even while reading nonfiction novels, the person a character fell in love with had smooth, radiant, glowing skin. Over time, I became my worst enemy and internalized society's mainstream idea of attractiveness based on what I've been seeing, reading, and hearing all my life. When characters that share similar physical features to you are continuously depicted as a hideous monster or "bad guy", it becomes so challenging to develop a positive self-image.

Feedback &

Criticism

I was walking from the guidance office with a friend and another girl walked pass us. As soon as she was a few feet apart, my friend commented "look at the bumps on her forehead". I didn't laugh because it wasn't funny. I didn't respond either because I didn't want to draw her focus onto me.

I asked my teacher to be excused from Algebra class to go to the restroom. Low and behold, I crossed paths in the hallway with a classmate who always picked on me. She was beautiful, and she looked me directly in my eyes. She remarked "breaking out are we" and laughed hoping to encourage others to laugh as well. I was speechless and felt the wind being knocked out of me. I just walked pass her and into the restroom, acting as though I didn't hear that cruel brutal comment. I cried so hard in the restroom. After about five minutes, I wiped my tears and came back to class walking with my head held high but still feeling mighty low.

I went to the campus café and waited in line. I saw this girl I knew and her friend. I spoke and gave her a hug. She squinted her eyes and said with disgust "why are all those bumps on your face?" She had flawless skin and her friend nudged her to keep her from being so rude. She seemed to care less about how that comment would have impacted me. I just looked at her with a blank stare, turned my head and walked away as if her remarks didn't even matter. When you have a meal plan or lunch in cafeteria, you have to eat what they're serving even when the only desirable items are greasy fries, pizza, fried chicken and hamburger. Those foods may not be the healthiest, but at least it kept me from starving at school; however, my body had a hard time digesting all that grease and oil. Eventually, the excess oil came out through the pores in my skin. My face continued to be ravaged by acne despite using acne medications.

While sitting on the porch with my grandma Lottie, I noticed she kept glancing at me looking very concerned. She said "what's wrong with your face, your skin?" I looked at her, got up and said "I don't know". That hurt! That was the most emotional painful experience I've ever had because at that point I felt powerless and very confused. I didn't have the answer to

her question. I left the porch and stood
in the yard for about 5 minutes. I felt
overwhelmed with sorrow because I was
causing her to suffer by just looking at
me. I returned to my seat and nothing else
was said about it. Later on, I looked into
the mirror and noticed that I had less acne
but my skin was so much darker, dried up,
and I literally looked like death. I took
myself off that Accutane medication. I
realized that sometimes feedback can
actually help us rather than hurt us. It
just may motivate us to make necessary
changes. When those medications write
"stay out of the sun", they mean it! The
warnings about the side effects are not to
be taken lightly.

During a Christmas gathering with the
family, a relative commented "I used to

have pimples on my nose too. You should put alcohol on that pimple so it will go down". I thought "was that a suggestion or a command". I put a dab of alcohol on my pimple, and it seemed to get bigger within the next couple of hours. I knew it wouldn't work, well not for me. However, I only entertained the idea so he leave me alone and wouldn't think that I wasn't trying to correct my skin problems.

I said to a female friend that I had a crush on, hoping to persuade her to look pass my appearance, "inner beauty instead of outer beauty should matter the most. Being understanding and smart with a great personality is what truly counts." She replied "somebody has lied to you. Being smart doesn't show up in pictures, only good looks". My response was "if they're

just good looking and not caring, good
looks won't show up when you in pain at the
hospital either. If you need a place to
stay, good looks alone won't offer to put a
roof over your head." Later that evening,
I began to think about my personal
experience. Most people would get "camera
ready" to take a picture with the finest
guy or girl at an event or party while the
average looking folks like myself are
pushed aside or go unnoticed.

There was an audition for a modeling
troupe on campus. I was actually attending
a seminar in the next room. From a
distance, two young female models were at
the door smiling and whispering. But as I
got up close, one remarked "never mind" and
turned her face in the opposite direction.
How rude!

My supervisor for my volunteer job thought I was having an allergic reaction on my face, breaking out in hives. She asked me "do you need a Benadryl?" I politely replied "no thank you, I'm fine." All a Benadryl will do for me is make me sleepy, and I will wake up looking the same. I laughed afterwards because I'm sure she didn't mean to offend me. Her skin was smooth, and it was clear to me she had never experienced skin issues.

It's so embarrassing to watch television with others and skin care product advertisements flash across the TV screen. It's even more embarrassing when they say, "have you tried that?"

It can be so annoying when someone says whatever you're using isn't' working. This medication worked on me and can probably help with your skin. However, what they fail to realize is that we don't experience breakouts the same nor will our treatment be the same.

I was walking through the mall one summer, and my face looked awful that afternoon. Unbeknownst to me was that the electronic store I was looking for was on the opposite end of the mall. The mall was so crowded, and I had to walk through the center. I was getting taunted by teens from both sides of the mall. Even adults were snickering at me. One girl even walked up to me and asked "would you like to be my boyfriend?" She laughed and went back to her circle of friends. At first, I walked with my head held high but as I continued to walk, it began to tilt downward. I felt humiliated. I finally

made it to that store and still had people
walking pass the store giggling and
pointing at me. There were times where I
found myself hiding behind the tape shelves
pretending to be tying my shoelaces.
However, I purchased what I needed and
departed at the nearest exit door. People
may view that experience as a tragedy but I
saw it as a victory. While I was walking,
I felt my knees getting weak and my eyes
getting watery. However, I continued to
press forward. I made up in my mind that
I've come too far to turn around and give
up. In spite of the many insults, I did
not allow the ridicule to keep me from
achieving my goal, making it to that store.
As I reflect on it, that shameful
experience turned into an unforgettable
lesson in life for me. My advice to you is

that you don't allow the criticism of others to keep you from enjoying life and pursuing your dreams. Folks will talk about you when you're looking good and will talk about you when you looking bad. As a result, you might as well be happy, move forward with your life, and not allow others to hold you back.

Overall, I've learned how to separate into categories people who give me feedback. If someone speaks to you about your skin out of concern because they care like my grandma Lottie, then be open to what they have to say. If someone asks questions out of curiosity because they don't understand, then try not to take it personal. However, if they make remarks just to be mean and hurt your feelings, then the feedback they give you should be

ignored and dismissed. Try not to allow
their negative opinions to become opinions
you form about yourself.

Mistakes I've made & Helpful Tips

Be careful where you pop your
pimples, in particular in public restrooms.
Make sure you don't touch surfaces and door
handles and then touch your face again.
You will be putting yourself at risk for
catching so many illnesses and germs. In
the moment, you don't really think about
the risks you're taking; at that point, you
just want to fix your skin problem not
realizing you may be inviting more health
problems in your life. Try to use a damp
paper towel instead of your hands to wipe
your face.

I try to avoid being around smoke
whether it comes from cigarettes, car
exhaust, or barbeque grills. Smoke can
clog up the pores in your skin and break
you out. I remember I attempted to smoke a
cigarette to deal with the stress of

breakouts and fit in trying to be cool.

However, it didn't help me relax but made

me more anxious and tense because I knew my

skin was going to rebel days later. As

predicted, my breakout was more severe. I

concluded that smoking is a habit I can't

afford to keep so I left it alone.

Try not to allow others to touch your

face with their hands, which may be full of

dirt, oil, or germs.

Read the fine print in those skin

product advertisements "individual results

may vary". Those companies usually just

showcase the success stories but some of us

that use those same products have tragic

endings. My motto is that product may be

proven to work for some, but it isn't

working for me. Find the skin care product

that's ideal for you, only if your skin has

not improved after a change in diet, sleep, stress level, or exercise.

Stress is not your friend. Do not allow yourself to brood and go to sleep angry at yourself. You've got to think positive and speak clear skin into existence, despite what you may be currently seeing in the mirror. With your mind, you are creating your days filled with either clouds of joy or misery.

Why are there huge mirrors everywhere at the gyms I've attended? I've noticed that men and women were not only checking out their bodies, but also their faces. They would get close up on the mirror and turn their heads from side to side. At least wait till you get to a restroom because people are watching you. If you're anything like me, you don't want to attract unwanted attention in your direction.

The longer you stare in the mirror, the more likely you'll find something in it that you dislike. Glance but don't stare for hours in the mirror.

We are taught to control our emotions. But trust me, its best that you acknowledge them and create an outlet for expressing them. If you don't, those bottled up feelings will come out and you'll lash out against yourself or someone you love.

I've dealt with skin issues by eating more sugary sweets. The more my skin broke out, the more sweets I ate, including cakes, pies, ice-cream, candy, gum, and chewy granola bars. I had so many dentist appointments; I didn't care. I knew that excess sugar was probably contributing to

my skin's poor condition, but I didn't care
because I was not willing to give up my
sweets. Until I watched Oprah Winfrey show
one day, and she was doing a segment on
overweight teens and stated "it's not about
the food, it's what you're hungry for".
That's when it hit me! Later that night, I
couldn't get that out of my mind. What was
I hungry for? It was control! I felt I
should be able to eat what I wanted without
my appearance being negatively impacted by
my diet. But the truth is that my
appearance worsened after eating too much
sugar. So my most important tip is to
watch what you eat and how it affects your
face. Greasy food and sweets (candy,
chocolate, cakes, sodas, juices with plenty
of sugar) can be your skin's worst enemy.
Important to note, when I significantly

reduced my sugar intake, my skin continued

to mildly break out but not nearly as bad

as before. As a result, I decided to take

another personal inventory of other foods I

ate. I realized I ate a bowl of cereal a

day. So I decided to limit the amount of

cheese or milk I ate. My skin has been

improving tremendously. Also, I left those

cooking oils and grease alone. I cook my

food in water and just season it really

good. Overall, you can control what you eat

but if you eat the wrong thing, you may not

be able to control how your skin will

react. I prefer prevention over

intervention any day of the week.

If you have to eat at a fast food

restaurant, use napkins to wipe off the

excess grease from the food. Some

waiters/waitresses got irritated with my

request for more napkins. However, I had to do what I had to do.

Also, don't allow pets to lick your face. Further, do not lay your head against their fur because it may be full of dust and dirt. However, continue to nurture your pets because they will love and accept you no matter what you look like.

If you put a skin cleansing face mask on the night before, sometimes the residue becomes deeply embedded in your skin. I've had green sparkles on my face the following day, and it wouldn't come off no matter how much I rinsed it. However, when I would exercise, it would come off as I sweated it out. So I advise you to exercise if you ever have a problem getting rid of the remains from a facial mask.

When pimples are clustered together

and you try to pop one that's not ready,
you'll just end up enlarging the others
that aren't ready either. At that point,
you'll feel even more exhausted and
frustrated. So if you feel that a pimple
is not ready to be popped, leave it alone.

Putting hand lotion or Vaseline on
your face after drying it out is not the
best route to take. I don't care who offers
you lotion to moisturize your face.
Mistakenly, I took a relative's advice,
applied their hand lotion on my face and my
skin exploded with pimples later that week.

Using acne medications and staying in
the sun for long periods of time is a huge
mistake. Even if you're using sunscreen,
I'll still advise you to stay out of the
sun. I am living proof and experienced the
awful side effects firsthand of mixing skin

care products with too much sunlight.

Putting alcohol on your face to reduce the size of pimples is not the best solution. Well for me, it had the opposite effect and increased the size of my pimples.

Try not to touch your face while eating greasy foods. I don't care how bad it may be itching. Find a restroom nearby, wash your hands thoroughly, and then touch your face if necessary.

Try not to worry about future breakouts, especially when there is a social event in the nearby future you're hoping to attend. Just enjoy each day and maintain your peace of mind with hopes that your skin will get better.

Be sure to get enough sleep at night. Sleep gave my face time to heal from everyday hardships. I try to sleep on my back so my face won't be pressed up against my pillow. Rarely do I sleep with my face down, only if I just washed my pillowcase.

I've tried to hide my face with the hats I wore. I used to depend on hats before I dared to go out in public. However, wearing hats can produce more heat. Where your hat rests, bumps may soon develop, especially on the forehead.

Too much sunlight can make your spots darker. With time, your natural complexion will return; just be patient and hang in there.

Wearing sunglasses can cause pimples to form on your nose. If you have to wear glasses, wipe them as often as possible. Also, if possible use a different rag and towel for your face and your body.

Don't allow others to physically fix
your skin with their fingers or hands. They
won't be as tender with your skin as you
would, and oftentimes make matters worse.

Be careful with your skin. There are
times to correct it and there are times to
leave it alone. Sometimes, it's best to
just let nature take its course.

Staying home and isolating yourself
from the rest of society is not always the
right answer for dealing with the shame of
having skin problems. My feelings of
sadness increased when I stayed trapped in
my room alone, away from family and
friends. You can still enjoy life and the
presence of others even if your skin is not
at its best. My good days in public have
definitely outweighed my bad ones.

Try not to wear a mask even on

special occasions. I wore a costume mask
during Halloween. My skin wasn't allowed to
breathe. I was sweating underneath my
mask. A huge pimple arose on my nose that
same week and other students criticized me.

When it's really windy outside and
dust/dirt is flying everywhere that dust
can slightly clog up your skin pores. Use a
damp cloth, and wipe your face once
indoors.

Don't put too much grease on your
head. You may want your hair to be shiny,
silky, and smooth. However, what you put on
top of your head, just might affect your
face. I choose not to grease my head at
all because when I did, my forehead was
full of small pimples. I even had them on
top of my head as well.

Find a mirror that highlights your

positive features and make you look beautiful. At work, I would walk pass several restrooms to get to the one that I looked best in. I would feel much more confident throughout the day. Dim the lighting if possible before you look into the mirror. Sometimes, you have to do what you have to do to feel good about yourself.

Every picture sparks an emotion whether it is good or bad. I would feel sad after looking at my pictures that showcased my bumpy skin. Pictures that I look bad in, I threw away. I needed to do what's best for me so I felt good at the end of the day. If a friend has a photo of us together, and I don't look good, I'll ask them to cut me out of that picture before putting me on their webpage or sharing it with others.

Some cameras or photographers can make you look beautiful while others don't portray you as being that cute. Find a good camera or photographer and know the distance the picture should be taken to capture your beauty. No close-ups please is my motto.

Watch how you hold your phone on the side of your face. Sometimes wax from my ears would get on my phone, and I would unknowingly rest it on the cheeks of my face. Later on, I would have bumps forming along the side of my face. So I advise you to not let the phone touch or rest on the side of your face.

When placing lip balm on your lips, be sure it doesn't touch the skin underneath or above the lips.

Washing your face constantly will dry

it out and make matters worse. Personally,
I don't scrub my face with a rag. I just
rub a bar of dove soap for sensitive skin
in my hands and gently caress my face.
Then I just rinse it off and dry it with a
clean towel.

What I want you
to learn from my
experiences?

Sometimes you may encounter an unwanted change in your skin that may catch you by surprise. Don't get frustrated; use that energy elsewhere. Next day, you'll feel better and realize you can handle this. It's not going to be easy, but you'll get through it. You know what you have to do; you can do it. You love yourself too much to be feeling down in the dumps. We're different because we've allowed others to have us feeling we are. There are other people that look just like us. There's nothing wrong with us. Just because we may have issues with our skin, does not mean we're not attractive. We're just as beautiful as everyone else. To the rest of the world, our skin may not be silky smooth and clear; however, as long as we feel that it's improving then that's all that matters. That should give you a confirmation that you're doing something right. You will be able to master your skin. Keep a journal of what you eat and be aware of how often you get stressed during the day. Find healthy ways to relax and laugh throughout the day.

It can be difficult to view ourselves as attractive when most of society feels differently. The belief system of what defines beauty for society was created before you were even born. You didn't adopt those belief systems overnight so don't expect to replace them in one day. It's going to take time to think new positive thoughts about yourself. However, it will be worth it and you'll find yourself feeling happier than you may be feeling right now. Try not to allow the

criticism of others to make you feel bad
about yourself. When you start
entertaining that, you're letting others
know that you value their input over your
own.

I was looking outside myself for answers
instead of unlocking the key to my beauty
which could be found through my
experiences. You know your skin better
than anyone else does. You be your best
doctor; you know what's working and what's
not. Don't put more faith in a product than
you do in your own inner wisdom gained
through your experiences. Those skin care
products may help a great deal, but not
cure acne; that's why they call it
treatment. You can be getting treatments
for the rest of your life if you don't eat
right, exercise, get enough sleep, and

learn effective ways to manage your stress.

In a society that values beauty that may be only skin deep, you'll have to learn how to be patient, forgiving and tolerant. Use your other gifts and talents to balance the odds that are against you. Love yourself even when others seem to be unable to look beyond what they see on the surface. As long as you're living, you are always in transition, and life will change for the better and so will your skin's appearance. Learn to love the skin you're in and if you have to decorate it with makeup or skin care products, then do what you have to do. As long as you feel good about yourself at the end of each day, then that's all that matters. Just realize, those products can only complement not compensate for the natural beauty that was there in the beginning.

Just always know that I love you, and you're not alone in your struggles with finding worth in your appearance.

About the Author

Howard Coleman Jr was born and raised in Fort Pierce, Florida where he attended Lincoln Park Academy High School. He moved to Tampa, Florida to attend the University of South Florida and currently residing in Tampa, Florida. He learned that changing your environment is great but changing how you see yourself is just as important. It took a while for him to find the courage to share his deepest feelings about his appearance. However, he wishes readers would find solace and comfort from his emotional pain during their own moments of insecurity about their appearance. Thank you so much for taking time to read this book and sharing with others that may benefit from it.

e-mail: howardjr2010@hotmail.com

Facebook: Howard Coleman

Instagram: howardcolemanjr

www.ingramcontent.com/pod-product-compliance
Lightning Source LLC
Chambersburg PA
CBHW070022260726
48658CB00009B/597